Ebola

I0448031

Lies

2.1

Exposing Lies with Documented Truth and How You Can Protect Yourself and Your Loved Ones

by JC Spencer

WHY EBOLA BECAME POLITICAL!

WARNING: Do NOT read this book unless you are open to verifiable truth that is disturbing.

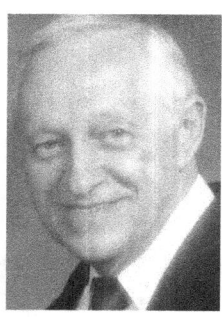

Author JC Spencer is CEO of The Endowment for Medical Research, Inc, a 501(c)(3) nonprofit, faith-based, medical research and education public charity and think tank based in Houston, Texas, which conducts nutritional surveys throughout the United States, Canada, and some foreign countries. For two decades, he has studied and conducted pilot surveys in the field of Glycoimmunology, a branch of Glycobiology.

He wrote the Glycoscience whitepaper -
www.Glycosciencewhitepaper.com

For details on booking the author for lectures at universities and fund-raising events contact him at
jcs@endowmentmed.org

Proceeds go to further education and research of Glycoscience through The Endowment for Medical Research, Inc., a 501(c)(3) nonprofit faith based scientific research, educational, public charity.

The Endowment for Medical Research
P. O. Box 73089, Houston, Texas 77273

www.endowmentmed.org

Content

Learn Hidden Ebola Facts

Preface

Overcoming the most lethal of viruses is one of the biggest challenges to face the human race. We are ignorant to many of Ebola's deceptive moves and the tricks and lies it has available to use against us. The information you will read in this book is alarming and can incite fear. My intent is to help others be informed and prepared for coming dangers.

Infectious diseases are not new but they are increasingly more deadly. Major plagues have killed millions of people in the past. The bubonic plague killed many millions of people in years gone by and it was a bacterium. Ebola is a virus and there are warning signs that it could become the worst plague in history.

Ebola started out as a nightmare for thousands. Ebola would soon cross oceans in a single bound, just a plane flight away. The global threat caught humans ill prepared and incompetent to respond beyond status quo. The plan is to fling billions of dollars against a wall of obstacles. Politicians, disconnected from medical reality, may do more harm than good as the embers of the most infectious epidemic smolder under cover of deception.

Deception and lies often miscommunicate what is really going on. However, today with all the communication technology available to us, IT IS MORE DIFFICULT TO CONCEAL TRUTH. Remember, TRUTH will always eventually prevail.

My desire is to help you learn how to protect yourself, your family and your immune system.[1] You have an important obligation to protect your family, those within your sphere of influence, and to bless and love others regardless of circumstances. The future is bright to those who open their eyes, confront the truth and become prepared.

The Ebola Zaire virus is the ultimate parasite - the worst of the worse. It can neither support nor propel itself. It cannot eat, secrete or reproduce on its own. Ebola is a skilled liar, deceiver and serial killer. And, you were told many **Ebola Lies**. The truth is amazing.

Introduction

Early on in my studies I was fascinated by a significant example of false communication which still causes so much havoc in the human body - the virus. The Ebola Zaire virus is the ultimate parasite that cannot support or propel itself. It can neither eat, secrete nor reproduce on its own. It is the ultimate liar, deceiver and serial killer.

I am going to plagiarize this Introduction to **Ebola Lies** from another book that is referenced in the back of this volume. The author should not mind. I wrote these following words about the virus several years ago.[2]

Viruses seize key positions on the surface of the cells. The virus is a key counterfeiter. Some viruses attack and disable their victims with cruel speed while others take years to harm their host. A virus, as in guerrilla warfare, can lie in wait for a more opportune time when your immune defenses are weakened.

The virus implements its evil plan by telling the cell, *"Don't reproduce yourself. Reproduce me. Here is my RNA to make yourself in my image."*

Let us look at a tiny *system*: If you think little tiny *systems* are not important, listen to the words of the Nobel laureate, professor Joshua Lederberg, PhD at Rockefeller University in New York City, *"Our only real competitors for dominion of the planet remain the viruses."*

A single virus is a tiny evil commando that cannot eat, secrete or propel itself. It is unable to reproduce without the aid of a living cell. The virus follows its preprogrammed instructions to reprogram the cells of another organism, making that organism its host.

By reprogramming the host cell, the virus causes that cell to become a traitor, directing it to cease its *designed function* and instead to replicate the invader, producing clones of the virus.

Stephen S. Morse, PhD and Robert D. Brown edited two books on the subject, Emerging Viruses and Evolutionary Biology of Viruses, where they said, "*The virus ... seizes key positions in the host's body and spreads to other hosts-in-waiting at the first opportunity. ... Some viruses attack and disable their victims with cruel speed. ... Other viruses take years to harm their hosts.* (HIV) *can incubate for up to a decade, allowing the deadly agent plenty of time to pass to new hosts before its ill-effects become apparent. Others* [viruses], *such as herpes simplex, coexist so well we're often unaware of their presence.*"

Some viruses mutate quickly. They do this by changes in the structure of their genetic material. In the virus, the RNA is actually changed. An ever-so-slight mutation of the antigens is all that is necessary to nullify all the antibodies that have been resident within a body for years. This enables the virus to sicken you all over again and again and again. Our bodies design a new antibody to go after the newly-*designed* invaders.

Morse and Brown conclude that "*if we don't take steps to monitor and contain their* [viruses'] *continual thrusts, one of their sorties could one day erupt into a global pandemic.*"

In 1994 Richard Preston wrote about the different strains of Ebola. He dedicated one chapter to Ebola Zaire and titled that chapter "*The Most Dangerous Strain.*" Ebola Zaire IS the current outbreak. If this virus gets outside a containment facility, it can devastate mankind. Ebola could go off like a forest fire. It is a Level 4 human hot agent and the reason for Preston's book, THE HOT ZONE.

Much appreciation goes to my wife, Karen, for her support, proofing, editing and suggestions to help make **Ebola Lies** more powerful and informative. I think that I have never written anything that she was not able to improve.   Thank you, honey!

Abbreviations

AIDS acquired immune deficiency syndrome
BMJ British Medical Journal
BSL-4 biosafety level 4 (highest level of danger)
CDC Center for Disease Control and Prevention Interest
CDC Center for Disease Control and Prevention Interest
CIA Central Intelligence Agency
DACA Deferred Action for Childhood Arrivals
DNA deoxyribonucleic acid - double helix - stores and transfers genetic information
DO - doctor of osteopathic medicine
DO - doctor of osteopathic medicine
DOD - Department of Defense
DOD - Department of Defense
DRC - Democratic Republic of the Congo
DWB/MSF - Doctors Without Borders / Medecins Sans Frontieres
EIS - Epidemic Intelligence Service officer for the CDC
EPA - Environment Protection Agency
FBI - Federal Beuro of Investigation
FD&C - food drugs & cosmetic dyes
GMO - Genetically Modified Organism
H1N1 - Swine influenza virus
HEPA - high-efficiency particulate air
HFCS - high fructose corn syrup
HIV - human immunodeficiency virus
Ibid - short for ibidem, citation for same as preceding footnote
ICE - Immigration and Customs Enforcement
INRB - National Institute of Biomedical Research /
    Instituto Nacional de Recursos Biológicos, I. P.
ISIS - terrorist group claiming Islamic State of Iraq and Syria
IRS - Internal Revenue Service
IU - International unit for measuring biological activity one = one mg
MAVNI - Military Accessions in the National
MD - medical doctor
MRSA - methicilln-resistant Staphylococcus aureus
MSF/DWB - Medecins Sans Frontieres/Doctors Without Borders
MSG - mono-sodium-glutamate
NIH - National Institutes of Health
NASA - National Aeronautics and Space Administration
OPA - Office of Population Affairs
PA - Office of Population Affairs
PhD - doctor of philosophy
RDA - Recommended Daily Allowance
RNA - ribonucleic acid - single helix, helps DNA make proteins from amino acids
sGP - non-structured glycoprotein
STD - Sexually Transmitted Disease
TB - tuberculosis
USAID - United States Agency for International Development
USAMRIID - United States Army Medical Research Institute of Infectious Diseases
UV - Ultraviolet light
WHO - World Health Organization

Ebola IS Out of the Bottle.

Can We Put the Ebola Genie Back in the Bottle?

The Ebola plague could bring more chaos and death to our planet than did the bubonic plague that killed millions in years gone by. Already, Ebola is an ember smoldering among the people awaiting the wind to ignite a fire that can only be resisted with a strong immune system.[3]

Medical personnel in multiple countries are testing positive after caring for those who have died of Ebola. Hundreds of health workers in West Africa have become infected where the death rate is 70% to 90%.

There are strong indications that some countries will be decimated. The World Health Organization (WHO) declares the end to an outbreak in a country when 42 days pass without a new case. Nigeria's 42nd day was October 20, 2014.[4,5]

Nigeria's surveillance remains on high alert. They understand the vulnerability from a new imported case. President Goodluck Jonathan has ordered continued vigilance at the nation's borders. Doctors Without Borders have played a significant role in helping stop Ebola in Nigeria.

The Center for Disease Control and Prevention (CDC), WHO and the US Army have not been on the same page.[6] The CDC in a futile attempt to be "politically correct" removed a Fact Sheet warning that Ebola can be spread by coughing and sneezing.[7] Denying all thoughts that Ebola is airborne, they even wanted to ignore that droplets are contagious. Meanwhile the WHO issued new guidelines for health workers that specify protective equipment should be worn to protect the mouth, nose and eyes from contaminated droplets and fluids. A U.N. agency said the new guidelines are based on a review of care of Ebola patients.

Removal of the Fact Sheet was another in a series of reversals. Does the CDC learn on the fly because of ignorance, neglect or cover-up? Finger pointing and not accepting responsibility is not new. The CDC blamed the Dallas hospital and two nurses who contracted Ebola from the first US Ebola case for not following their guidelines. The CDC insisted their protocols were sufficient; but, that statement was shot dead when they issued new guidelines while continuing the stance that there is no risk of Ebola airborne transmission. At the same time, the US Army published its seventh edition of its medical management handbook that warns viral hemorrhagic fever, the category of viruses that includes Ebola, can be an airborne threat in certain circumstances.

We have a plague that may be aided by political deception.

When is Ebola Contained?

Ebola is contained by keeping the infected from the uninfected. Ebola was naturally contained years ago because it was so lethal that it killed every man, woman and child in the village before they could travel to another village. Today, you can circle the globe faster than a village citizen can trek to a distant village.

An unusual characteristic of this Ebola epidemic is a pattern of persistent cyclical dips in the number of new cases, followed by sudden flare-ups. The virus may become latent for decades before it breaks out again. Its longevity is unknown. Ebola can always return at a more opportune time.

The WHO said the number of deaths estimated in Africa is probably three times the number earlier quoted. The WHO also acknowledged the Ebola epidemic continues to accelerate in Guinea, Liberia and Sierra Leone. They declared the outbreak ended in Senegal on October 17 and in Nigeria on October 21, 2014 because of no new cases within a 42 day period.

The Fatal Flaw in the Ebola Test

There is a fatal flaw in the Ebola test.[8] The test does not become positive until the symptoms have manifested for a few days. An infected person will test negative until there is viral buildup in the body. Dr.

Nancy Khardouri, director of infectious disease at Eastern Virginia Medical School, has studied and treated infectious diseases for the past 30 years. She says the test is a main concern.

The world saw the results of this flawed testing with the first New York City Ebola patient.[9] Dr. Craig Spencer was the first person in New York City to test positive for Ebola.[10]

German Doctors Provide Evidence

German doctors provide evidence that Ebola can be transmitted BEFORE the patient has the symptoms.[11] There is a high risk of acute infection from contact with bodily fluids, such as blood, sweat, vomit, feces, urine, saliva or semen. It was previously believed that those fluids must have an entry point, like a cut or scrape or someone touching the nose, mouth or eyes with contaminated hands, or being splashed.

Contamination can occur by touching an infected doorknob or surface. Touching the face with contaminated hands can increase the risk. A hand shake, cough or sneeze can transmit Ebola before the transmitter ever develops a fever. The incubation period for Ebola seems to be from one to three weeks or more (7 to 21+ days). As the number of infections increases, so does the export possibility that a person with Ebola will carry it to another country. Some scientists are now indicating that the incubation period may be longer - up to 42 days.[12]

What about Ebola Survivors and Sex?

The virus has been found in semen and vaginal fluids of survivors.[13] The knowledge that Ebola can survive months after symptoms of Ebola have abated has triggered concern that the virus could be spread via sexual contact with otherwise healthy individuals. One study found that Ebola remains active in semen for 90 days. US health officials are resounding this caution as the survivors are released back out into the public with the suggestion to only engage in protected sex.

Twenty-nine people recovering from Ebola in the Congo were part of a 1999 study. Four of the five recovering patients and their households (including sex partners) were observed for up to 21 months. None of the 29 sexual partners had symptoms of Ebola although four of the five patients tested had at least one semen sample with the Ebola virus.[14,15]

Daniel Bausch, knows Ebola personally perhaps better than any American doctor today. He was director of the Emerging Infections Department at the U.S. Naval Medical Research facility in Peru and he is a professor at the Tulane School of Public Health and Tropical Medicine. He has been to West Africa several times.[16]

It's difficult to know when a virus is dormant. Can it become active again? Studies by Bausch and others detected the Ebola virus in sexual fluids that grow in cell culture. Scientists question if it is possible that sexually transmitted Ebola may have flown under the radar for lack of data from the outbreaks in past years. As with any infectious disease, patients with a high viral load in their fluids obviously increase the risk to others. It is difficult for the Ebola virus to exit the body. This may result in the virus remaining in the body even after it appears to be cleared from the blood.

Dr. Bausch believes the current outbreak to be much worse than ever before. He helped assemble the medical teams. Ebola has decimated the leadership that he put in place. Dr. Sheik Humarr Khan the veteran chief physician at the Kenema Clinic whom Dr. Bausch hired ten years ago and had worked side-by-side with him, died from Ebola in July 2014.

At one point Dr. Bausch thought the Ebola fire was almost out. It had been contained, he thought, but later said, "*You can't put out 99 percent of a forest fire - you have to put it all out.*"

A virus is an evil stealth killer and will lie in wait for a more opportune time to strike with the force to wipe out millions. Our obligation is to be prepared for the next outbreak. There will be the next outbreak!

Mutation

The secondary infection rate was observed by Ira Longini, a biostatistician at the University of Florida. This study evaluated how many get the Ebola virus from an infected person in relationship to previous outbreaks. This may provide evidence of possible mutation of the virus and whether it has become more transmissible. Mutation could allow the spreading of Ebola to remain active longer, become more violent or become airborne.

Today, many experts scoff at the possibility of Ebola mutating into an airborne virus. However, back in the 1980s, General Dr. Philip Russell expressed concern and declared that everyone at USAMRIID (US Army Medical Research Institute of Infection Diseases) "*concluded that Ebola is airborne.*" Colonel Nancy Jaax who confirmed that the Zaire Ebola in a monkey was exposed through the lungs in 1986. "*There were Ebola crystalloids bursting out of the lungs... The lungs were popping Ebola directly into the air.*"[17]

The CDC has continued to deny that Ebola is airborne. Confusion with mixed messages abound. However, Purdue University Professor of biological sciences, David Sanders, believes it can mutate to be airborne if it hasn't already. In fact, one of the five strains of Ebola has mutated and is airborne: that is Ebola Reston (not involved in the current outbreak). In 1989 this strain was discovered in Reston, Virginia and could be spread through the air, Sanders explained. Interesting, is the fact that the Ebola Reston does not seem harmful to humans. Yet, under the microscope it appears identical to Ebola Zaire.[18]

BEYOND Ebola is Already Here

Epidemic infectious diseases are already here. The CDC reminds us that sexually transmitted diseases (STD) are a hidden epidemic. Today, 110 million in the US have STDs (50.5 million men and 59.5 million women). Influenza is #7 of the 17 leading causes of death in the US.[19] The influenza pandemic of 1918-1919 was considered the most devastating epidemic that killed more people than World War I. The WHO's Global Tuberculosis Report 2014 confirms that TB remains the second greatest infectious disease killer, infecting about nine million people last year, killing 1.5 million. Pandora's box of drugs is not much hope. Hope for resistance to infection will be found in better sanitation habits, more cautious behavior and strengthening of the human immune system.

Mathematical Calculations

Mathematical calculations favor the triumph of Ebola once it gains a foothold.[20] Global health officials are looking closely at the "*reproduction number,*" in West Africa which estimates how many people will be infected by each person stricken. A recent analysis projects the number at 1.5 to 2. The epidemic will begin to decline when that number falls below one. Meanwhile, the outbreak in West Africa is unprecedented.

Viral speed is much faster than bureaucratic real time. Cases in Africa are doubling about every three weeks excluding the countries where Ebola has been contained. There is indication that for every two known Ebola cases three more are not reported. Ebola propagates in mucous membranes that makes contamination easier and more likely.

The WHO warns that West Africa can soon face up to 10,000 new Ebola cases a week.[21] The head of the CDC warned that the Ebola virus could become a global calamity on the scale of HIV.

The CDC predicts, at the current infection rate, that Ebola could infect up to 1.4 million people within three months.

Canadian researchers have discovered that monkeys can catch Ebola from infected pigs without coming into direct contact. Now, we have humans with Ebola who were not in direct contact with an Ebola patient. More mysteries about Ebola keep appearing.[22]

Doctors Without Borders

Note: Medecins Sans Frontieres (MSF) is the medical charity known in English as Doctors Without Borders.

We have reports that 22 of its staff were infected with Ebola and that 15 have already died. Their website in October 2014 stated they have treated *"around 3,200 confirmed Ebola cases and around 1,200 have survived."* According to their figures more than 2,000 have died of Ebola.

A spokesman for MSF stated that their staffs were

issued personal protective equipment that includes, among other things:

- Cape
- Gloves
- Rubber surgical apron
- Surgical trousers and tunic
- Rubber boots
- Respirator mask/face protector
- Hood
- Wrap-around goggles / Antifog spray

The total cost is approximately $90. Some of the protective gear is sanitized and reused and some wearable items are used once then destroyed.

Juli Switala, a South African pediatrician with MSF, explained that her team had to make difficult decisions to not resuscitate babies out of fear that the staff may be infected. The outbreak is devastating Guinea, Liberia and Sierra Leone.

Lucey said, "*I don't see a light at the end of the tunnel. The epidemic is still getting worse.*" Lucey is a physician/professor from Georgetown University.

The MSF has offices in 28 countries, and in 1999 MSF won a Nobel Peace Prize for its humanitarian services. The money was used to study neglected diseases.

New York City's First Confirmed Ebola Case

Dr. Craig Spencer, with Doctors Without Borders, recently returned from Guinea. This is the 4th patient in the US and the first in New York City diagnosed with Ebola. Three of the four are doctors returning from Africa where they were treating Ebola patients.

A city spokesperson said officials are attempting to track all of his contacts including a trip from Manhattan to Brooklyn on three subway lines and a visit to a bowling alley.

The doctor returned to the US within the presumed 21 day incubation period. The report said Dr. Spencer worked in emergency medicine at New York-Presbyterian Hospital/Columbia University Medical Center, and taught at Columbia University.

It is confirmed that the doctor cleared the newest enhanced screening protocols when he returned from Africa through JFK Airport on Oct. 17. He went through multiple layers of screening and did not have a fever or other symptoms of illness.

Consequently, for those returning from an Ebola country, the CDC adjusted the protocol for 'post-arrival monitoring' by state and local health departments to 21 days after returning from an Ebola country. The incubation period is 21 days but some health authorities put it at 42 days. They confess that Ebola is proving to be a tricky pathogen to spot in patients who appear well. Many Americans have lost confidence in the CDC's ability to contain Ebola.

Untrained city workers after having contact with the infected Dr. Spencer, removed their protective suits, touched the outside of the suits and discarded them in public trash cans. It appears the CDC guidance from our government medical professionals was unbelievably derelict.

Ebola is Biosafety Level 4 (BSL-4)

Experts in infectious diseases, microbiologists, immunologists and epidemiologists, are alarmed at the procedures and lack of precautions used to protect the US from Ebola. Doctors, aid workers and military personnel can be in serious danger when they use BSL-3 equipment in a BSL-4 situation.[23,24]

Ebola is declared a Biosafety Level 4 (BSL-4) pathogen. Level 4 is the highest virulence designation for infectious agents. Ebola Zaire, the strain that's gone wild, is considered the worst of the strains. The CDC in a 59 page document explains the significance of these 4 levels.

Effective BSL-4 personal protective equipment is flexible, impenetrable material and a high-efficiency particulate air (HEPA) filtration system designed to filter out viruses. There is profound concern for the thousands of US military personnel who are not wearing BSL-4 gear while working with Ebola patients. Pictures confirm that personnel are wearing

Biosafety Level 3 (BSL-3) protective equipment made from Tyvek suits, paper face masks and a face shield that's open at the bottom. Tyvek is tough material but easily punctured by any sharp object. Should any contaminant splash onto a paper mask, the wearer will most likely breathe the contamination.

Reports indicate that precautions are inadequate. Health workers have been hit hard by the virus. Doctors in Spain scrambled to protect individuals at risk after a nurse was infected with Ebola. A UN worker died of Ebola in a German[25,26] hospital despite "*intensive medical procedures*." The St. George hospital in Leipzig said the 56-year-old man tested positive for Ebola on Oct. 6 and died a week later, prompting Liberia's U.N. peacekeeping mission to put 41 other staff members under "*close medical observation*." This gave rise for concern in Europe.

Congo Reports New Ebola Cases

Reports coming out of the Democratic Republic of the Congo (DRC) are sketchy but the WHO estimated 62 cases of the Congo Ebola outbreak. The death rate in the Congo is 90%.

A team of national and international specialists have been deployed to the Congo to work with the local response teams. Patients are being treated in temporary isolation units in Watsi Kengo, Lokolia, Boende, and Boende Muke. A mobile laboratory from the National Institute of Biomedical Research (INRB -

Instituto Nacional de Recursos Biológicos, I. P.) has been installed in Lokolia and is currently functional. Two laboratory epidemiologists from the US Centers for Disease Control and Prevention have arrived in DRC to support the INRB field team.

Ebola appears under control in the Congo. The WHO may declare the country Ebola free after 42 days without a new case. Recently, 49 people have died in the Congo with the last confirmed case of Ebola in October 2014.

Since the July 2014 outbreak of Congo Ebola, reports are that the Obama administration has brought into the US at least 1,900 refugees from the disease-stricken nation who have been resettled in the US, according to statistics provided by the State Department.[27]

The Congo Ebola strain is slightly different from the virus that has been ravaging West Africa. Researchers have concluded the Congolese outbreak is not connected to the epidemic in West Africa. It is believed that eating contaminated animal meat started the outbreaks.

The Bureau of Population, Refugees and Migration's report shows 944 refugees were admitted from the Congo in July; 628 in August and 338 in September, for a total of 1,910 Congolese refugees during these three months of 2014.

The US refugee program is on schedule to resettle 70,000 citizens, including a limit for the fiscal year of

2014 of 14,000 from Africa.

The report documents the US has given priority to Congolese refugees, as we joined the United Nations and international resettlement community to resettle 50,000 Congolese over the next few years.

A Summary of Bad Choices which Makes the World More Dangerous Today

- The CDC recently, AGAIN, lost vials of bird flu viruses, anthrax and other highly pathogenic materials. They totally disappeared with no record of where they went. Did these highly dangerous pathogens fall into enemy hands?

- The first Ebola patient's family in Dallas was left in their apartment with bloody sheets for three days. Government officials know that Ebola spreads by contact with bodily fluids.

- Infectious bodily fluids were pressure sprayed into the air and flushed down the Dallas city drain. Some vomit may have been eaten by a dog which can be infected.

- The CDC director said that it would be counterproductive to cut off air travel from the Ebola infected nations.

- US borders are intentionally left wide open. Border patrol agents report that illegal aliens are entering the US with serious infectious diseases. During the first seven months of 2014, it was reported that at least 71 confirmed undocumented immigrants came across our borders from Ebola outbreak nations.[28,29]

- FBI Director said that we can't stop Americans who are fighting for ISIS or other terrorist groups from re-entering the country. This is unbelievable since they have declared war on the US.

- The Ebola epidemic in West Africa started in February 2014. The CDC put in place the protocol and training of medical personnel eight months later.

- An Ebola Czar with no medical experience was appointed. He has stated his thoughts for population control especially in Africa and Asia.[30,31]

- Terrorist or stupid robbers? Bandits stole a cooler bag of Ebola infested blood from a Red Cross courier in Guinea. Was the blood the target or a terrifying surprise for the bandits?

"Ebola Jihad"

Ebola Jihad[32] has been declared on America by ISIS and other terrorist organizations. They intend to purposely infect people and fly them into the US. Reports are that terrorists have been arrested at the Texas border. Wrong is called right, bitter is called sweet, darkness is called light, lies are called truth and bad choices continue to come in waves. Political correctness and Executive Orders change neither diseases nor the laws of physics.

3 Reasons for bad choices

The three reasons for all bad choices are ignorance, neglect and rebellion. When all three happen at the same time, it is probably political.

Not having the right knowledge, neglecting to act on right knowledge or consciously choosing what is known to be wrong makes right choices impossible.

Many scientists and world leaders are on record espousing population control as the solution to solve the planet's problems. Hmmm?

Population Control

I recall a natural disaster in Bangladesh that killed

100,000 people. An official's response still rings in my ears and sends chills up my spine, "*The monsoon was a failure. It only killed 100,000.*"

Global population reduction policies are taught in our universities and espoused by globalists.[33] The idea is to reduce the world's population by 2 billion people in any way possible. Some have gone as far as to openly recommend that homosexuals, poor people, blacks and those who are not productive (the elderly and disabled) be targeted.[34,35]

This Policy is endorsed by the US State Department's Office of Population Affairs (OPA), established in 1975 by Henry Kissinger. This group drafted the Carter administration's *Global 2000* document, which calls for global population reduction and the policy constitutes conscious depopulation projects.

The globalists believe development programs have created a population time bomb. This is their rationalization for reducing the population by 2 billion people. They believe that if there were no population control there will be civil war and greater food shortages because there are just too many people on the planet. The globalists blame themselves for letting people breed like flies, for increasing the survival rate, for extending life and for lowering the death rate. They consider it their own failure for not reducing the birthrate earlier. So drastic action is now required which helps explain the massive push for abortion.

Famous people in high positions of government and finance claim that the "*population crisis may be a greater threat to national security than nuclear annihilation.*"[36]

When hygiene is less than adequate, infection is more rampant. The Ebola outbreak rages in West Africa and experts believe it is destined for Asia where billions of humans are crowded into ever more confining areas.

From the personal experiences which I have had in Africa, India and the Middle-East, I attest to the fact that the hygiene is inadequate. In fact, the conditions are ripe for the largest genocidal event in world history whether perpetrated by war or Ebola.

Ron Klain, Obama's Ebola Czar, has no medical experience but he has stated that one of his biggest fears is "*overpopulation especially in Asia and Africa that lack the resources to have a healthy, happy life.*" Klain added, "*And I think we've got to find a way to make the world work for everyone.*"

Some individuals will continue to influence foreign policy based on a genocidal reduction of the world's population. "*We have a network in place of cothinkers in the government,*" said the OPA case officer. "*We keep going, no matter who is in the White House.*"

Bio-weapons are a reality and if Ebola were used in a jihad scenario, it should be treated akin to a nuclear attack on the US. A Missouri physician accuses the CDC of dereliction of duty with Ebola.[37] "*It's reactionary, not responsive.*" Dr. Gil Mobley is a microbiologist and trauma physician in Springfield,

Missouri. He returned from a medical mission trip in Guatemala and was not asked any questions upon re-entry into the country other than whether he had alcohol or cigarettes. When he came through Customs: *"They didn't ask me where I'd been. They didn't ask me if I'd been sick. They didn't ask me if I'd had a fever. And they didn't thermo-scan for my temperature."* This was after the Ebola case in Dallas.

A microbiology expert with 30 years experience, Dr. William Miller, author of the pioneering book, <u>The Microcosm Within: Evolution and Extinction in the Hologenome</u>," said that the establishment is on the wrong side of medical science and is playing Russian roulette by keeping our borders porous. Dr. Miller explained that the plan will inflict a suicidal wound on US.

Were Pogo and Chicken Little both right?
"We have met the enemy and it is us."
"The sky is falling! The sky is falling!"

But wait, the war is not over! Deception will be exposed and truth will set us free.

Why Ebola Became Political

Politicians have stressed that you cannot let a crisis go to waste. Instead of solving the crisis, too often the response is: *"What can we get out of it."* The more mass confusion created, the more the public is willing to yield control to the politicians. A viral pandemic is most effective in creating a domino effect for control.

Statesman and Senator Ted Cruz (R-TX), says the US Ebola policy "*seems to be dictated by politics rather than a common-sense approach to protecting the American public*."

Donald Trump speculated that there's "*something seriously wrong with President Obama's mental health*" for refusing to cut off flights to countries with active Ebola cases. Trump added, "*He's either incompetent, he's very stubborn or there's something wrong.*"[38]

Dr. Ben Cason says that we should fear martial law. President Obama and most of the politicians and bureaucrats evidence more concern about political power, wealth and their own selfish desires than they do about our country and its citizens.

Bad political strategy uses the uninformed, the ignorant. The uninformed are played for fools for votes gained with meaningless words. Ebola may be the ultimate crisis they cannot let go to waste. Ebola could be the perfect "*act of nature's crisis*" to make the failures of man seem insignificant.

Obama's own administration sees that he is willing to sacrifice them. Instead of promised transparency, he spews a steady stream of lies, egregious violations of our laws, obstructions of justice, victimizing, spying, decimation of the military, flagrant disregard for our Constitution, targeting those who disagree with him, aiding terrorists, illegally swapping five terrorists for a presumed traitor, gun grabbing, gun running, treason and now aiding Ebola and ISIS.

We have already seen whole industries threatened or destroyed by Executive Orders. But, perhaps the scariest: Obama quietly gave himself the power to impose martial law, bypassing both the Constitution and Congress through Executive Order. Executive Order No. 13603, the *National Defense Resources Preparedness Executive Order*, gives him extraordinary powers. Many believe a manufactured crisis could be in his mind to permit him to bring about socialism to America, allow him to create a powerful regime and declare himself a supreme dictator over all the land.

When leaders double down on propaganda that is clearly illogical and untrue, the citizens cannot and should not have confidence in their words. Misrepresentations and nebulous assurances that all possible precautions are used to combat the spread of Ebola raise suspicions because the words and actions are not congruent.

Add chaos to chaos. The quarantined Nurse Kaci Hickox who refused to remain quarantined misled the press. She apparently worked with Doctors Without Borders caring for Ebola stricken individuals in West Africa. However, records indicate she was an official CDC Epidemic Intelligence Service officer. According to the *Daily Caller*, Hickox was listed as an active EIS officer as of July 2014, per CDC documents. Her actions, as a CDC Epidemic Intel officer, underlined how unimportant it is to the CDC to take adequate precautions. The CDC actually issued the statement, *"Returning Ebola medical workers should not be quarantined."*[39,40]

Clearly it has been determined and demonstrated that political expedience trumps public concerns. Our problems cannot be solved politically. Politics is a symptom. We have learned that treating symptoms instead of the problem will cure nothing. The problems in America are spiritual and moral.

Decoy - Deception - Destruction
How Ebola Accomplishes its Dastardly Deeds

We learned HOW Ebola functions by observing the destruction. Here the dying Ebola patients gave us the answer!

Deceive the Generals with a Decoy
With only seven genes, the Ebola virus writes scripts to rival a Hollywood murder thriller. The frontal attack is to disable the immune system generals including the macrophage, killer T cells and other white blood cells. To disable the warriors that are in charge of foreign enemies is a masterful military tactic if you are invading a country. Once the generals have been set aside, Ebola can run lawlessly throughout the whole body.

Soldiers are Dismissed
and Their Weapons are Taken
Structured glycoproteins on the surface of healthy cells give life to the cell. An army of an estimated

800,000 glycoprotein receptors sites are on the surface of each healthy human cell. These antennae receive and transmit communication and process DNA data. Each cell has an army of these defenders that make up the communication system for the immune system and every function of the body. The only hope against sickness or any virus is a well equipped, well armed, healthy immune system.

Scientists report that the Ebola virus instructs the infected cells by editing the RNA to produce and secrete non-structured glycoproteins (sGP) into the blood stream.[41,42,43,44] These broken down glycoprotein snippet pieces appear to serve no function other than as decoys to confuse the immune system.

Wounded Warriors Become Totally Defenseless
The fewer glycoproteins on the cell the sicker the cell. The infected cell grows weaker as the glycoprotein structures are dismantled.

Healthy cells fight off infection and communicate the need for hydration and nutrients. When Ebola attacks, the cells immediately begin to dehydrate.

The Glycoprotein warriors have multifunctional benefits beyond the communication for the body. One function is to occupy all the docking stations on the cell so viruses will not be able to attach to the cell in the first place. The Ebola virus has a difficult time destroying healthy cells. The weaker cells succumb.

Ebola causes the blood and water of the body to act strangely. They are no longer congruent. Neither the blood nor water can travel to where they are needed. The blood coagulates and does not flow properly and the water and waste become diarrhea. According to doctors at Emory University Hospital and from other reports, Ebola patients produce diarrhea at the rate of 1½ to 3 gallons (5 to 12 liters) per day.[45,46]

With the rapid dehydration go essential minerals and electrolytes required to power the mitochondria which soon overheat and bring about the fever. The body's destruction is complete within days.

An interesting side note: *One of the important sugar building blocks of the glycoprotein structure is the mannose molecule, which is scientifically known as mucilaginous polysaccharide because of its mucus texture. This feature makes the blood cells slippier and able to better circulate throughout the body.*

How Big of a Health Crisis Can Be Created or Allowed to Happen?

Much in common:
Ebola and Terrorists

Governments have engineered biological weapons for decades. Weapons of mass destruction have been found in Iraq and are now in the hands of ISIS. Captured fighter jets are in ISIS's hands in northern Syria. Many believe the missing Malaysian Airline plane is also in terrorist hands. Eye witnesses have observed training of pilots as they conduct take-off and landing exercises at the Aleppo airport where it is reported that ISIS captured the jets. It is only a few minutes from there to Israel.

Now, we see the merging of biotech warfare with terrorist activity while some "leaders" actually believe it is part of the answer to benefit the planet. A viral pandemic will be rationalized as necessary for the greater good of the masses. Any objection to government action will be labeled as evil and perhaps subjected to punishment. The public will agree because fear controls, which in turn, propels the uninformed into the arms of tyrants. Terrorists have become a serious health problem.

It Depends on What IS IS

It is often ever-so-difficult to tell the good guys from the bad guys. Nothing is as it appears. The public is shocked and horrified at human acts that kill anyone anywhere. When we see brothers fighting, we have compassion and want to help. But, it may not be wise to step in (even if we have the best intent to keep the peace). Conniving brothers who have been fighting for years, may be luring you into the fight so they can turn on you.

Here is the way it is working, intended or not. We arm the "moderates" who then surrender to the radicals. By this method, the US is arming Al Qaeda, ISIS and other terrorists.

Other evidence that we are funding barbarians is that we, that's US, have subsidized and continue to subsidize militant extremists. In this case our government leaders consider other groups of terrorist "freedom fighters." Because some groups of barbarians share a mutual enemy with us, we help fund their actions with about 1½ million tax payer's dollars PER DAY.[47]

Some time ago, Obama considered the solution to peace in the Middle East would be to utilize the Syrian Free Army - a group Obama had earlier referred to as "fantasy" and just a bunch of "doctors, farmers, and pharmacists." Former U.S. Marine Corps 34th Commandant General James T. Conway stated the strategy doesn't have a snowball's chance in hell of succeeding.

Drinking the political cool aid has resulted in complacency, inaction and wrong decisions that have compounded the Ebola War. The struggle is to blame anyone or anything except self. An attempt to shift the blame for man's failures to "God did it" will not succeed but for a season.

To Fundamentally Transform US

We do not learn from politicians by what they say. Listen not to their words but observe what they do. In order to fundamentally transform the US as Obama promised, he simply needed to change the purpose of government agencies and implement regulations to impair growth. More government is increasingly more incapable of protecting the people.[48]

Credibility is a sacrifice that must be made to accomplish an evil objective. Removal of credibility from each agency is part of the plan. Others are busily focused on the many targets of incompetent agencies and people. The public becomes angry and wants them gone. We have witnessed people with such evil determination that they are willing to virtually blow themselves up to achieve the goal.

A few examples: The new mission for NASA is relationship building with Muslims. The Environmental Protection Agency (EPA) chokes progress and tramples over property rights of citizens in the name of environment. I am all for protecting the planet for our health reasons; but, a lizard should not triumph over a human's well being. Politicians make slaves out of the poor so they are more dependant on an incapable government. The corrupt IRS is now ordered to oversee healthcare. The CDC seems more focused on mandatory motorcycle helmet laws, playground accidents, video games and violence than they are on Ebola. So, Ebola is relegated to the military.

First Time in US History

For the first time in US history there is a new Military program for illegal immigrants[49] known as *Military Accessions in the National Interest* (MAVNI). This program is open to immigrants without a proper visa if they came to the US with their parents before age 16.

Illegal immigrants without proper visas are scheduled to be approved under a 2012 Administration policy known as *Deferred Action for Child Arrivals.* Misleading the public even more, illegal children approved under DACA can be as old as 31 years of age. Based on an honor system, anyone claiming to be a part of the program cannot be deported.

The plan outlined by the Department of Defense will allow illegal aliens to join our military and receive citizenship. Already, 90,000 real soldiers and officers serving in our military have been fired leaving room for possible infiltrators. It is criminal to arm an illegal person, but laws do not seem to matter.

The Army's 101st Airborne Division is one of the most highly decorated fighting units in the US Army trained for air assault operations. Why was this Division and others called into the Ebola War poorly equipped to handle the situation?

Estimates indicate that more than 4,000 US forces are expected to be deployed to West Africa. It was declared that the mission was to build treatment facilities and train healthcare workers; but, almost all of the initial military deployment are some of the nation's top combat-trained troops.[50]

Since World War I, the 101st has taken part in historic military campaigns, including leading the D-Day night drop campaign prior to American airborne landings in Normandy. The force's central roles include the Battle of the Bulge, wars in Vietnam and the Persian Gulf, first and second Iraq wars and the US war in Afghanistan.

There's no room for conspiracy theories, just truth. Too often instead of asking hard questions, the media attempts to discredit the messenger. Without question, Ebola is dangerous. It is illogical to think otherwise. Still, reports abound with myths and misconceptions.

US Army veterans, including US Army Generals want facts not fiction. It is reported that Generals who have expressed their views have been silenced.

Jessica L. Write, undersecretary of defense for personnel and readiness, identified three levels of training. Level II training will be for personnel who "*interact with the local populace*," and Level III training is for personnel "*assigned to supporting medical units or expected to handle exposed remains.*"

If the troops are required to complete Levels II and III of training, the instructions are opposite to previous public statements from DOD that those deployed will not be exposed to Ebola but will only serve a "*supportive role.*" But, that changed too. A volunteer group of our troops will be taking care of the infected medical personnel.

We have been assured that our military personnel would not be in direct contact with Ebola patients.

However, it appears that promise is another deadly lie. A DOD memo outlines new training for our troops to have direct contact with "exposed remains" of Ebola victims. The memorandum, on page 19, in an attachment summarizes this training.

According to Dr. Daniel Bausch, if an Ebola patient's dies, his or her viral load at death is particularly high, which boosts the risk of contracting the disease from interacting with the corpse.

The health concerns are that our troops will be exposed to the virus, bring it to the US and potentially destroy the US military along with much of the population. If I were the enemy, I would salute those who made this decision. Now, let us look at the final directive the troops receive just before departure to West Africa.

Prior to departure, all military personnel will receive immunizations for hepatitis A and B, tetanus-diphtheria, measles, polio virus, seasonal influenza, varicella, typhoid, meningococcal and rabies. ***GOD, PROTECT OUR TROOPS***!

Take a penny and look at it. Read the statement on that little copper plaque, **IN GOD WE TRUST**. Now, put the penny back in you pocket and keep it close to you. The statement on the coin is priceless. Treasure it!

Vaccines Raise Serious Questions as More Lies are Revealed

On the surface it looks like the CDC is protecting our troops. Rabies? These immunizations are risky and very serious. From the list for hepatitis A and B, tetanus-diphtheria, measles, polio virus, seasonal influenza, varicella, typhoid, meningococcal and rabies, let's take a quick look at what may be the mildest vaccine - the influenza shot.

A *Johns Hopkins University School of Medicine* scientist, Peter Doshi, Ph.D., charges that influenza vaccines are less effective and cause more side effects than alleged by the CDC. The paper was published June 2013 in the British Medical Journal (BMJ). Doshi says that the studies do not substantiate the official claims made by the CDC. The marketing tactics of the drug companies are well planned and aggressive. Twenty years ago, 32 million annual doses of influenza vaccine were available in the United States. In 2014 at least 135 million annual vaccine doses go into our population.[51]

Doshi further states that the CDC is lying about the high risk of flu complications which can cause death. That's *"not the case,"* said Doshi.

In people with a good immune system, the risk from the flu vaccination is greater than the flu. Doshi further stated, *"This means that influenza vaccines are approved for use in older people despite any clinical trials demonstrating a reduction in serious outcomes,"* says Doshi.[52]

An Australian study that found one in every 110 children under the age of five had convulsions following vaccinations in 2009 for H1N1 influenza. Additional investigations found that the H1N1 vaccine was also associated with a spike in cases of narcolepsy among adolescents.

Dr. Russell Blaylock, a neurosurgeon is on record that *"Not only is the vaccine not safe, it does not even work. The vaccine is completely worthless, and the government knows it."* Continuing, he says. *"The government also says that every baby over the age of six months should have a vaccine, and they know it contains a dose of mercury that is toxic to the brain. They also know the studies have shown that the flu vaccine has zero* - zero - *effectiveness in children under five."*

The fact is that for many people, the flu shot depresses the immune system especially in children. Many people have expressed concern that the flu shot gave them the flu.

Mercury affects the brain for several years and some neurologists believe it may be the cause of Alzheimer's and other degenerative diseases. Dr. Blaylock reported that one study found that those who get the flu vaccine for three to five years increase their risk of Alzheimer's disease 10-fold.

Vaccines fulfill pharmaceutical dreams for making billions of dollars with full protection. The US Congress passed a Law that no one can sue a pharmaceutical company for side effects from vaccines even though they are complete frauds. The National Childhood Vaccine Injury Act of 1986 was upheld by the Supreme Court in 2011 in a court ruling of 6 to 2.

It looks like the only real inoculation is given by our Congress. This was a real shot in the arm for the pharmaceutical companies.

There is evidence that the formulation for some vaccines contain a birth control ingredient which may be used in population control. One of several documents on vaccines and population control are available in the US National Library of Medicine at www.PubMed.gov.[53]

Various means are used to weaken our military. There is clear evidence that the influence is coming through the Muslim Brotherhood within the Pentagon. Recently the career of Lt. Col Matthew Dooley, a West Point graduate and highly decorated officer, was destroyed. He was teaching the course, *"Perspectives on Islam and Islamic Radicalism"*.[54,55]

Chairman of the Joint Chiefs of Staff, Martin Dempsey has publicly degraded and reprimanded our military leaders through negative Officer Evaluation Reports. Col. Dooley has now been added to the 9 Generals the administration has summarily dismissed.

Richard Thompson, of the Thomas More Law Center said, "*All US military Combatant Commands, Services, the National Guard Bureau, and Joint Chiefs are under Dempsey's Muslim Brotherhood-dictated order to ensure that henceforth, no US military course will ever again teach truth about Islam that the jihadist enemy finds offensive, or just too informative.*"

Former CIA agent Claire M. Lopez *(about Lt. Col. Dooley)...*" *The ... Administration has demonstrated lightning speed to dismiss military brass that does not conform to its agenda, and not surprisingly, nobody is speaking up for Lt. Col. Dooley.*"

The question begs to be asked, "*Why have 197 Senior Military Commanders been dismissed in five years including 9 Generals in 2013?*"

NEW Army of Violent Criminals Freed from Jails

This could affect your health. Newly released documents reveal that hundreds of illegal immigrants charged with violent crimes and serious felonies have been released from jails across the country.[56]

The Immigration and Customs Enforcement agency has now admitted that numerous dangerous criminals have been released but denied any direct responsibility.

According to records obtained by USA Today (October 2014), the government has released inmates charged with offenses ranging from kidnaping and sexual assault to drug trafficking, armed assault and homicide.

The evidence contradicts previous assurances by the administration that the 617 criminals who were released as part of a cost cutting exercise were low risk offenders charged with misdemeanors "*or other criminals whose prior conviction did not pose a violent threat to public safety,*" USA Today reported.

The administration released an army of more than 2,200 illegal immigrants from jail between Feb. 9 and March 1, 2013, as part of an effort to cut the number of prisoners due to the budget sequester funding cuts. The detainees were waiting deportation or immigration hearings in a court, and the administration did not give advance notice it would be freeing them.

Texas, Florida, Massachusetts, Colorado among other states have recaptured illegal immigrant criminals and charged them with use of weapons, kidnaping, sexual assaults and murder.

The releases triggered a furor in Congress. Hearings with lawmakers grilled John Morton, then Director of Immigration and Customs Enforcement (ICE).

According to USA Today, Virginia GOP Rep. J. Randy Forbes asked Morton directly, "*No one on that list has been charged or convicted with murder, rape, or sexual abuse of a minor, were they*?"

Morton, who subsequently resigned, answered with a lie, "*They were not.*"

Former White House spokesman Jay Carney had also described the criminals as "*low-risk, noncriminal detainees*," USA Today reported.

Meanwhile, Republican Sens. John McCain of Arizona and Tom Coburn of Oklahoma demanded a formal investigation by the Inspector General. "*It is baffling how an agency charged with homeland security and immigration enforcement would knowingly release hundreds of illegals with criminal histories. In this single action, ICE undermined its own credibility, the rule of law, and the safety of Americans and local law enforcement*," Coburn said when the audit was released.

Senator McCain said it is "*deeply troubling that ICE would knowingly release thousands of undocumented immigrant detainees - many with prior criminal records - into our streets, while publicly downplaying the danger they posed*," USA Today reported.

It is baffling unless you realize we are at war.

To unleash a tidal wave of illegal border crossings with overwhelming law enforcement and give a "*free pass*" to the cartels. The President by unconstitutional executive orders undermines the rule of law and make law enforcement an impossibility. That is the plan?

Top sheriffs across the country are bracing for Obama to release another army of criminals on the US. Every county in America will become a border county. Paul Babeu, Sheriff of Pinal County, Arizona is quoted as saying, *"The law applies to you and I as citizens, and yet it appears there is no law when it comes to illegals."*

Sheriff Chuck Jenkins of Frederick County, Maryland believes, *"... based on what I've seen, every county in America will become a border county."* We will see an increase in criminals coming into our country. There will be an increase in crime, infiltration of gangs, drug trade and human trafficking.

Sheriff Sam Page of Rockingham County, North Carolina said, *"Human trafficking, drug trafficking and criminal activity are coming through our borders, but not staying near our borders. It's getting into every part of the US."* TB, dengue fever, hepatitis, malaria, measles and Chagas diseases will be unleashed.

Chagas is life-threatening. Chagas is caused by protozo found in 21 Latin American counties and affecting some 18 million people. Physician Dr. Elizabeth Lee Vilet has been involved with medical projects in Central and South America since 2009. Her article, *"Deadly Diseases Crossing Border with Illegal Immigrants"* was published in June 25, 2014. Illegal immigrants from Latin America are bringing diseases to the US that we had under control or had nearly eradicated, including TB, dengue fever, hepatitis, malaria, measles and Chagas diseases.

100,000 Haitians

Now, comes 100,000 Haitians without visas, fraught with medical risks from outbreaks of cholera and the chikungunya virus. Haiti has the highest incidence of HIV and AIDS infection for any country outside of Africa. Report are that more than 715,000 people in Haiti, the Dominican Republic and Cuba have been sickened by cholera. Nearly 9,000 have died from cholera. Haiti is ravaged by the chikungunya virus with a recent report of 27,541 cases in the country. Yellow fever outbreaks have resulted from mosquito infestation.[57]

An estimated 100,000 Haitians are approved to arrive in the US under the reunification program. They are awaiting visas. A branch of Homeland Security (US Citizenship and Immigration Services) announced it plans to expedite a program to reunite Haitians already living in the US with family members abroad. Sounds compassionate but this could result in the deaths of many innocent Americans.

Some on the Senate Judiciary Committee, warned that this was likely just the beginning of unilateral and executive actions on immigration. The CDC has failed before to provide proper medical screening prior to arrival. Will this massive error be corrected?

Economic Impact

The Ebola War goes beyond what will effect human health. Ebola will compound the economic problem for many countries and the impact will become global. Tipping a domino is easy. The world economic system is already "one sick puppy." The central banks are out of control and fueling a bubble that is about to burst.[58,59]

A Lesson for US

A clear lesson for the US is to observe similarities between Ebola in Nigeria and other places. Ebola was the same but management determines totally different outcomes.

The difference between a disastrous outcome and conquering the enemy is determined by: (1) how quickly we correct the stumbles; (2) how we properly diagnose; (3) have sufficient training; and (4) have supervised defense. Fast and thorough tracing of all potential contacts must be ongoing. Monitoring of all of those exposed is vital along with rapid isolation of potentially infectious contacts. Hopefully, we have learned to put better safety protocols in place.

The Weapon of UV Light

The Ultra Violet light spectrum renders the DNA/RNA in bacteria and viruses impotent to reproduce. In other words, UV light kills Ebola dead.[60] UV light should be used as a weapon in the hands of every health worker.

For many years, scientists have observed that certain specific light spectrums have beneficial or harmful attributes. The US National Library of Medicine has on file a 1982 paper showing that the Ebola virus and other viruses are made inactive by gamma irradiation.

Ebola is a complex virus with interesting characteristics. One beneficial factor is that it is more sensitive to UV light and therefore easier to kill with UV radiation than other viruses. A paper published in 2007 shows that replication and transcription of Ebola's RNA genetic codes are fused beyond recovery with UV light.

A group of doctors in Texas has developed the Xenex Germ-Zapping Robot that kills the Ebola virus with UV light. The RNA or DNA is rendered unreproductive. The robot uses three different types of ultraviolet light. The first two, UV-A and UV-B, are part of the spectrum that reaches the surface of the Earth. The third, UV-C, is blocked by the Earth's ozone layer, and organisms have no defenses against it. The $100,000 Xenex germ killer uses xenon gas to create UV-C light that is 25,000 times more powerful than natural sunlight. The Robot is already in use in 250 hospitals.[61]

How Shall We Then Live?

The ultimate answer for your body to be able to resist or fight any disease is the strength of your immune system.

The treatments for Ebola in most cases involve nothing more than the steady replacement of vital fluids, electrolytes and plasma until the patient's body can build up an immunity to the virus.[17] Those with stronger immune systems before contraction of Ebola are more likely to survive and beat back the disease. Survival depends on how you respond and take care of your immune system.

You can lead by example by focusing on educating yourself on how to strengthen your immune system and improve your overall health. Teach and promote healthy hygiene and sanitation habits to those you love. Local grass root groups including doctors and healthcare professionals working together and supporting each other will provide community strength through a common sense approach.

We cannot count on government to help us. It is government who needs our help. The talent and technology of our citizens are available to make our nation strong and safe.

The spread of Ebola prompted the US Agency for International Development (USAID) to launch *"Fighting Ebola: A Grand Challenge for Development"* initiative on October 7, 2014. Solicitation of ideas can be used to improve the equipment available to African health workers treating Ebola patients on the front lines, particularly as they operate in hot, humid environments that make impermeable suits very difficult to wear. President Obama announced the initiative at the Global Health Security Summit in Washington, D.C., and his administration has said they want to field any new innovations within months.

What do I do next?

Of course, if you have had any contact with anyone who may have been exposed to Ebola, consult with your healthcare professional.

The most important health benefit any of us can accomplish is to **STRENGTHEN OUR IMMUNE SYSTEM!**

The Building Blocks of Your Immune System

There are several important pathways to naturally support your immune system but one provides the BUILDING BLOCKS OF OUR IMMUNE SYSTEMS!

These building blocks are necessary sugars, yes sugars! But, they're really unusually beneficial sugars, vital to the very existence of our lives and well-being. These sugars structures naturally coat every cell of our bodies are actually antennae that provide the signaling for everything that happens in our bodies. To have a healthy body and strong immune system, it is essential that these building blocks be complete. I will cover these functional, biological sugars at the end of this next section.

Natural Ways to Improve Your Immune System

A good immune system is not only based on what you DO but on what you do NOT DO! A healthy lifestyle starts with a decision. It's your choice.

Avoid Foods, Beverages and Ingredients that Cause Inflammation

Most chronic conditions like cancer, arthritis, diabetes and obesity have been linked to inflammation. Inflammation is a factor in most health issues.

Table Sugar - The *American Journal of Clinical Nutrition* warns that table sugar and other high-glycemic starches increase inflammation. Especially harmful is high fructose corn syrup (HFCS) and artificial sweeteners which weaken your immune system and cause other health challenges.

Trans Fats - Back in the 1990's, Harvard School of Public Health researchers started teaching that inflammation is triggered by trans fat that is found in most fast foods, fried foods, processed snack foods, donuts and margarine. Stay away from products that have ingredients of **hydrogenated or partially hydrogenated oils** - these are bad trans fats. It really does pay to read labels!

For cooking and baking, educate yourself on the healthy oils such as extra virgin olive oil and coconut oil.

Omega-6 Fatty Acids - The average American gets more omega-6 fatty acids in their diets than omega-3s which causes an imbalance that can lead to inflammation, according to U.S. News. Cut back on omega-6 found in heavy seeds and vegetable oils. Consume more fatty fish and walnuts.

Food Additives - Artificial colors, chemical additives, synthetic flavor enhancers, stabilizers and preservatives are harmful. Some of the main ones include sulfites, benzoates and colors. The worst dyes for health include Food Drugs & Cosmetic Dyes (FD&C) Blue No. 1, Blue No. 2, Green No, 3, Red No. 3, Red No. 40, Yellow No. 6 and Yellow No. 6. Unfortunately, many foods consumed by children are loaded with these harmful, toxic ingredients are used in ice-cream, soft drinks, dairy products, and canned foods.

MSG - Many people discover that they have **gluten** intolerance. That problem may be triggered by **MSG (mono-sodium-glutamate)**. I have written about how MSG can open the sodium ion gates of cells to absorb the glutamate which can affect the DNA. MSG can cause chronic inflammation and liver problems.

Soft Drinks contain high fructose corn syrup (HFCS), sugar or harmful synthetic sweeteners such as Nutrasweet, Splenda, saccharin, aspartame and other harmful additives that weaken the immune system.

Alcohol, even in "moderation," (less than thought) can cause inflammation of the liver and brain. What's best for the body? Pure water.

Make it a habit to switch out the no-so-good food and drinks for natural, healthier replacements. Let it become a game. Make it fun. But, eating right is more than a game. It's a matter of a less painful and longer life because you reduce inflammation in your body.

White foods
Many **white foods** are harmful. White flour products, white potatoes, white rice and white table sugar are all known to stimulate inflammation.

Switch out the white potato for a sweet potato. Believe it or not, the sweet potato is lower glycemic and more healthy for you. The glycemic index is based on how quickly a food converts to glucose in the body. The white potato is high glycemic. High glycemic foods turn quickly to glucose. You can lower the glycemic index of the white potato with lots of butter and sour cream which may not be the right choice for other reasons.

White table sugar is not the best choice but that

which replaces it may be even worse. **Aspartame** (Equal) is a neurotoxin that can cause inflammation that affects the brain. It would be wiser to replace the sugar in your sugar bowl with **Trehalose**, a healthy sugar. It may make a world of difference in your health. I explain how regular table sugar causes some 145 health challenges. Researchers have published papers on 65 significant health benefits especially neurological benefits of Trehalose.[62]

The book, **Change Your Sugar - Change Your Life** can be downloaded at www.DiabeticHope.com I reference many of the studies with Trehalose and its ability to keep the cells hydrated.[63,64] The sugar Trehalose strengthens the cell membrane and has significant benefits in protecting human cells from extreme conditions. Much research is needed in relationship to Ebola.

GMO foods

A genetically modified organism (GMO) is an organism whose genetic material has been altered using genetic engineering techniques.[65] Organisms that have been genetically modified include micro-organisms.

Make every attempt to stay away from GMO foods that not only can cause inflammation, but a hosts of other problems in our bodies. Jeffery Smith in Genetic Roulette outlines 65 health risks from GMO foods. He says that gene insertion disrupts the DNA and can create unpredictable health problems. When genes are inserted at random into the DNA, their location can influence their function, as well as the function of natural genes. Altered gene expression is serious.

One study using a micro-array gene chip found that 5% of the host's genes changed their levels of expression after a single gene was inserted. These changes can have multiple health-related effects. They can overproduce toxic chemicals in the cell or block function of other genes. GMO foods can actually aid viruses to splice themselves into the host's DNA. The instability of inserted gene material may create many unpredicted effects. Mutations to animal and human offspring can manifest for generations to come.

Take Positive Action Now

Put color in your life
Right eating includes plenty of greens plus colorful vegetables and fruit with antioxidants to combat free radicals. Free radicals damage the DNA and lowers your immune system.

Water, more water
Drink plenty of water and avoid soft drinks. Even so-called energy drinks can add to infection. Lots of good clean water flush toxins out your system. Very few people drink enough water. Water is essential to carry waste out of your body. And, a good home filter produces water much purer and less expensive than bottled water. And, the water actually tastes good! If you don't use a filter; you become a filter.

Improve blood circulation

Your immune system is improved through your blood. Without proper circulation, inflammation happens. Life is in the blood and circulation of the blood nourishes every cell of your body.

Adequate exercise is probably more that what you are getting. We need to move more, stretch more, do more. To climb stairs is a good exercise. A study was conducted of sedentary, elderly, healthy people. The researchers were surprised that all of them lived in two story houses and climbed stairs.

An interesting study was reported in 2006 where researchers took 115 obese, sedentary, postmeno-pausal women and assigned half of them to do stretching exercises once a week and the other half to do at least 45 minutes of moderate intensity exercise five days a week. At the end of this year long study, the stretchers had three times more colds than the moderate exercise group.

Stress less

Chronic (long term) stress is tough on your whole body including the immune system. Stress causes your adrenal glands to pump adrenaline and cortisol into your body which over time taxes the immune system raising the risk for viruses and hyper-reactive immune responses.

Many of us need to learn how to better relax and save our stress responses for emergencies. Meditation is wonderful for the immune system when it is on that which is good, true, honest, pure, lovely, good and virtuous. Quiet music has proven to be effective for producing positive changes in the immune system. Studies have indicated that the sugar Trehalose relieves cell stress, is a mild antidepressant and provide sustained energy to the body.

Proper sleep
Sleep allows our bodies to rest and repair. Lack of sleep is a real culprit in weakening the immune system. Sleep deprivation depresses the immune system and elevates inflammatory chemicals. The men and women who habitually slept less than seven hours a night were almost three times more likely to develop a cold than those who slept eight or more hours.

Shun tobacco smoke
Linda B. White, M.D. reports that one of the ways to strengthen the immune system is to shun tobacco smoke. She says that tobacco smoke triggers inflammation, increases respiratory mucus, and inhibits hairlike projections inside your nose (cilia) from clearing that mucus. Children and adults exposed to tobacco smoke are more at risk for respiratory infections, including colds, bronchitis, pneumonia, sinusitis and middle ear infections.

Hygiene
To keep down infection and possible inflammation in the body, it is vital to maintain clean hands and body, inside and out. Wash your hands for 15 to 20 seconds preferably with hot water and good soap before meals and after coughing, sneezing, using the restroom or touching surfaces that may be unclean.

Supplements that support the immune system
We do not get the nutrients in our processed foods that our grandparents did. It is important to supplement our food with quality products that are made from food, not chemicals, to provide the missing nutrition.

Food Sourced Vitamins and Minerals
Governments require ingredients in the bottle of nutrition be listed on its label. But, if the nutrients are not absorbed into your cells, what difference does it make? Ninety five percent (95%) of vitamin supplements are made from coal tar or petroleum products. Most mineral supplements are made from rock or metals. They say they are all natural and that claim is correct. But, when you can still read the name on tablets drudged from the city sewage plant, you know the absorption rate is quite low.

Vitamin D
Dr. Linda B. White also writes about the importance of the roles that **Vitamin D** plays in promoting normal immune function. She explains: "*Vitamin D deficiency correlates with asthma, cancer, several autoimmune diseases (e.g., multiple sclerosis), and susceptibility to infection (including viral respiratory infections). One study linked deficiency to a greater likelihood of carrying MRSA (methicillin-resistant Staphylococcus aureus) in the nose.*

"Unfortunately, nearly one-third of the U.S. population is vitamin D deficient. Because few foods contain much vitamin D, your best bet is to regularly spend short periods of time in the sun (without sunscreen),

and to take supplements in northern climes during the colder months. Guidelines for the Recommended Daily Allowance (RDA) of vitamin D, currently set at 400 IU/day, are being revised. Experts predict that the new RDA will be about 1,000 IU/day (25 ug/day)."

Our opinion is that anyone not getting enough sun exposure, should supplement with a good quality natural Vitamin D.

Probiotics

Also, a very important supplement for maintaining a healthy immune system is **probiotic** bacteria.

Dr. Mercola is a DO (osteopathic physician) who is also board-certified in family medicine trained in both traditional and natural medicine. As he points out, *"Most people, including many physicians, do not realize that 80 percent of your immune system is located in your digestive system, making a healthy gut a major focal point if you want to maintain optimal health. Remember, a robust immune system is your number one defense system against ALL disease."*

He believes that most people have an imbalance in their digestive system which is *"the nutritional root of so many health concerns."* Dr. Mercola reports that *"A new study shows that probiotics can modulate immune responses via your gut's mucosal immune system. It was found that probiotics have an anti-inflammatory potential. They caused a decrease in serum CPR levels, and a reduction in the bacteria-induced production of pro-inflammatory cytokines."*

Unsweetened yogurt (you can add fruit or sweetener when you eat it), some cheeses and sauerkraut are good sources of natural, healthy bacteria. A high quality probiotic supplement is often needed as well to adequately populate the intestinal flora.

A Brief Response -
WHAT ARE SMART SUGARS?

For two decades, Smart Sugars have been our focus. Smart Sugars are the building blocks of your immune system.

The term, Glycobiology was coined at Oxford University in 1988. Glyco is Greek for sugar and Glycobiology is a branch of biology which deals with sugars. Scientists have identified about twenty-seven bio active sugars found in nature that I call Smart Sugars. Here is a brief look at a few of these Smart Sugars. More information is available in the book, Smart Sugars.

- **Mannose:** Studies show that mannose has remarkable health benefits, especially involving the immune system, cognitive functions, and cancer. Your god health depends on it. Mannose is cited by the National Library of Medicine in more than 27,000 research references linked to studies.

- **Fucose:** (not to be confused with fructose) Fucose, with major health benefits, may prevent and treat cancer. The National Library of Medicine cites more than 9,700 research references with more than 1,400 linked to cancer studies.

- **Trehalose:** Trehalose has a clean sweet taste that other Smart Sugars do not have. It can be used instead of table sugar. Trehalose is able to protect the integrity of cells against a variety of environmental stresses such as dehydration, heat, cold and oxidation. Trehalose has an important functionality that aids in the proper folding of proteins. More than 6,000 research references are cited by the National Library of Medicine. Trehalose helps hydrate cells. The sugar Trehalose strengthens the cell membrane and has significant benefits in protecting human cells from extreme conditions. Much research is needed especially in relationship to Ebola.

- **Galactose:** Studies reveal significant galactose health benefits: Babies are dependant upon it to build their immune system and help structure the glycoprotein receptor sites. More than 33,000 references cited by the National Library of Medicine.

- **Glucose:** The medical establishment recognizes the basic sugar glucose as very important to human life. However, it appears to be the most harmful in large quantities, especially for diabetics. Glucose is often used as an intravenous drip in hospitals.

Researchers are giving Smart Sugars serious exploration. More physicians are beginning to incorporate these sugars into their practice by asking their patients to eat them. More individuals are ingesting these natural sugars and discovering health benefits. Drug companies are rushing to synthesize these sugars into new drugs. Many thousands of patents related to these super sugars have been issued, especially since 1995.

We are presently aware of a small but growing number of very significant super sugars. Eight of these sugars were presented by Robert K. Murray, MD, Ph.D., and published in multiple editions of <u>Harper's Biochemistry</u>.

Here are some of the sugars that I consider Smart Sugars, part of the Royal Family of Sugars:

Fucose,	Galactose,	Trehalose,
Glucose,	Glucosamine,	Xylose,
Galactosamine,	Sialyllactose,	Arabinose,
Mannose,	Lactose,	Ribose,
Rhamnose,	N-acetylgalactosamine,	

N-acetyl-D-N-acetylneuraminic acid
N-acetylglucosamine.

The benefits have become self-evident and scientists have concluded that super sugars have efficacy individually and synergistically that build cells, coat cells, strengthen cells and cell membranes and aid in the cell manufacturing of glycolipids and glyco-proteins.

Glycoscience is the future of medicine. Some 800,000 transmitting sugar antennae coat each healthy human cell resembling little bushy trees. These antennae are constructed from mannose, fucose, glucose, galactose, xylose, N-acetylglucosamine, and variations of other Smart Sugars.

Each antenna is a glycoprotein or glycan. A glycan is a tiny tree-like structure of these different sugars linked together. A glycoprotein is made of sugar and protein links. Without glycans, the cell cannot live. These glycans actually give us life and intelligence. Without these sugars the human cell would have no life.

Become educated in the facts and take action on your newly found knowledge to better your health. The Endowment for Medical Research offers, as a public service, more free educational material. The general public and healthcare professionals are invited to study our websites that could take hundreds of hours to peruse.

Healthcare professionals and the general public have free access to the Glycoscience whitepaper at www.Glycosciencewhitepaper.com

---

The Source and Reference section at the end of this book is not exhaustive on the subject and students are welcome to study our educational websites for more comprehensive studies.

www.GlycoscienceNEWS.com and
www.Glycosciencewhitepaper.com

Additional reading and training materials

Available worldwide on Amazon or in our
Bookstore: www.endowmentmed.org

Read this book and learn
WHY WE SHOULD LISTEN!

Smart Sugars
Sugars that Speak.
Why we should listen!

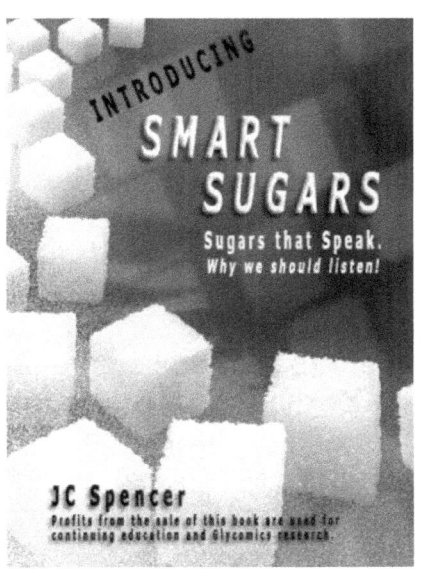

An introduction to Glycoscience. Easy to read for the student while packed with new information for the seasoned medical professional, research scientist, and learned professor.

Smart Sugars is *NOW* available in Hardbound, soft cover, Kindle and in Audio

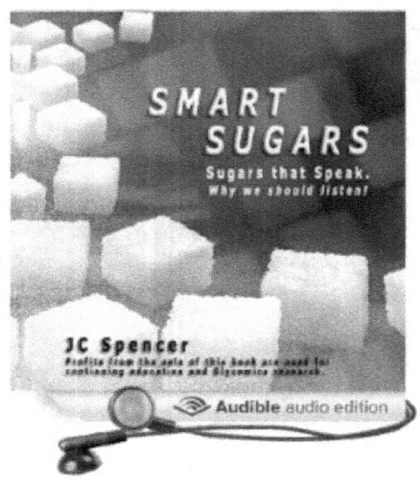

Smart Sugars

[Unabridged]
Audible Audio Edition

by JC Spencer (Author),
Ross Merrick (Narrator)

Listen on your Kindle Fire or with the free Audible app on Apple, Android, and Windows devices.

Cut and paste Link below to listen to a video sample of the reading of Smart Sugars
www.SmartSugars.com/audio or
http://www.amazon.com/Smart-Sugars/dp/B00OI2H6VW/ref=sr_1_sc_1?ie=UTF8&qid=1414528141&sr=8-1-spell&keywords=Smart+Surgars+audio+book

Editorial Reviews on Amazon

Smart Sugars is an easy to read book about the breakthrough of sugar technology that will change the way we live. The author explains that some 800,000 transmitting antennae called glycans (actually sugar) coat each of our healthy cells like fuzz on a peach. **Smart Sugars** will help us take the focus off of the disease, treat and cure, because of these new discoveries. Tomorrow's doctors will use Glycoscience diagnostics to read our cells to better determine health and what our health will or can be years in advance.

Available on Amazon in softback for only $3.77
Go to www.Amazon.com and type in **Enjoy Smart Sugars**

Enjoy Smart Sugars

We have conclusive documentation that we can improve brain function with certain sugars.

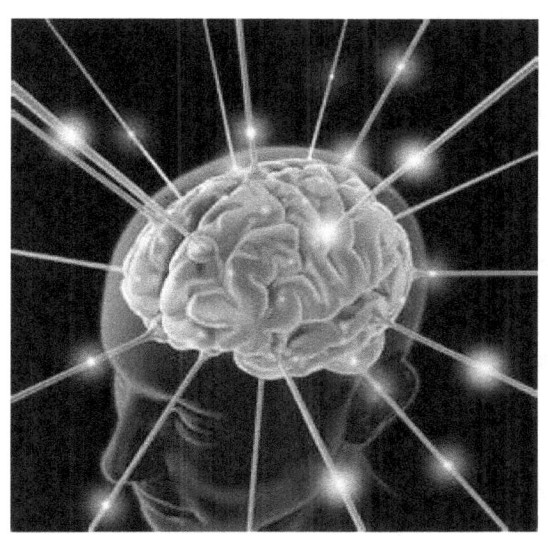

This book is your guide to help you improve brain function, overcome stress, and become healthier.

You may wish to participate in a pilot survey.

This is not a booklet of ideas. This is an ACTION book and the next step is up to you.

This Glycoscience textbook is for the learned scientist and inquisitive individual.

Expand Your MIND - Improve Your BRAIN
is an easy to read entertaining 580 page science book.
This textbook references over 700 MDs, PhDs, Scientists,
Researchers and Educators in the field of Glycomics and Brain
Function.

Available Three Volumes in 1 or Volumes 1, 2, and 3 Separately.

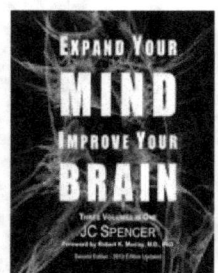 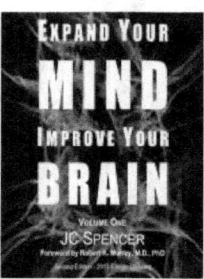 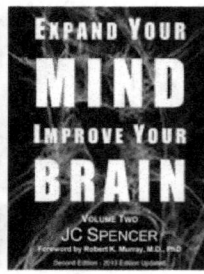 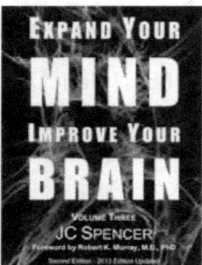

First Edition published in 2008
Second Edition - 2013 Edition - Updated. Available as an e-textbook, perfect bound 8 1/5 x 11, and hardbound editions

Three Volumes in One
          Softbound .... $ 77.77
          Hardbound $127.77

Vol. 1; 2 and 3 individually as ebook only . $ 27.77 each
      or 3 Volumes in One e-textbook ...... $ 47.77

Order in the Book Store at www.endowmentmed.org

This is an educational project of The Endowment for Medical Research

101 Smart Sugars Lessons that clearly present the progress of Glycoscience and where it will take us.

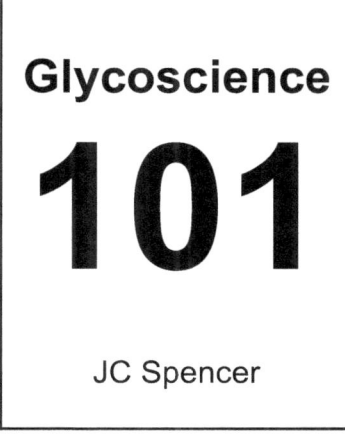

The Trehalose Handbooks are available 3 Volumes in 1 or Volume 1, 2 and 3 Separately.

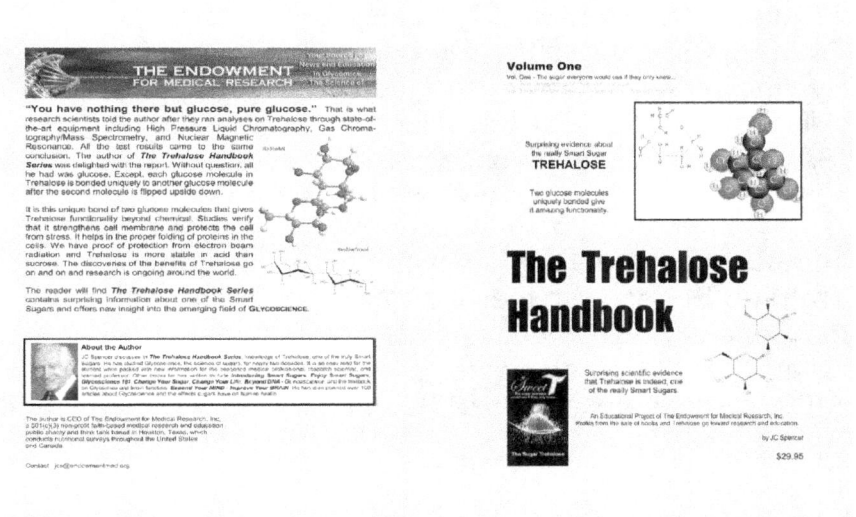

Available in the Book Store at
www.endowmentmed.org

Video Training for the Healthcare Profession and for the General Public.

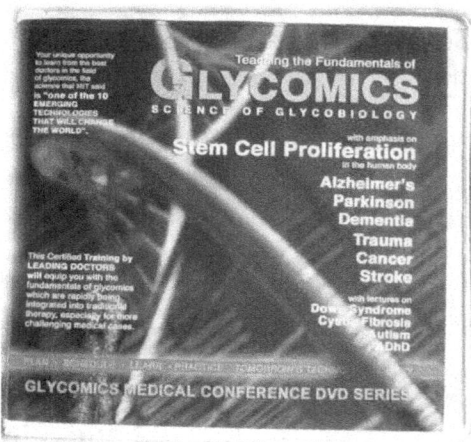

14 hours Professional Glycomics DVD Video Training Series from the Glycomics Conference for Healthcare Professionals. Included is a 500 page syllabus on CD plus all the color slides presented (SAVE $100 off regular price of $299) $199

(Testing available)

14 hours General Public Glycomics DVD Video Training Series from the Glycomics Conference for the General Public (does not include 500 page syllabus of all the color slides presented (SAVE $100 off regular price of $199) .... $ 99

For details on booking JC Spencer for lectures at universities and fund raising events contact him at jcs@endowmentmed.org

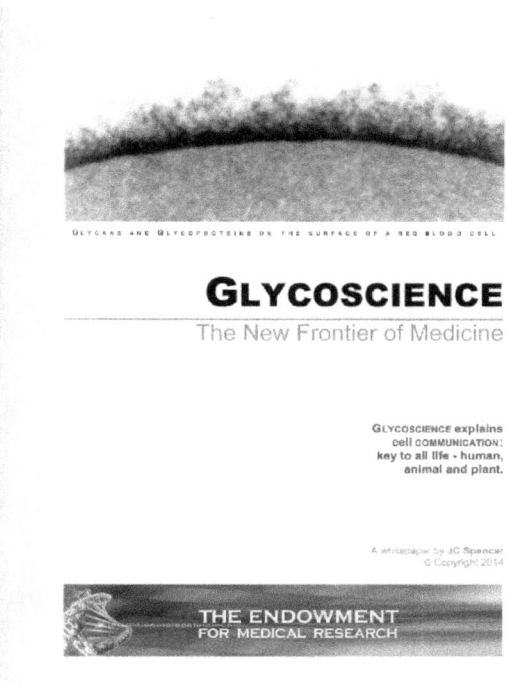

GLYCOSCIENCE

The New Frontier of Medicine

GLYCOSCIENCE explains
cell COMMUNICATION:
key to all life - human,
animal and plant.

A whitepaper by JC Spencer
© Copyright 2014

THE ENDOWMENT
FOR MEDICAL RESEARCH

The authoritative Glycoscience whitepaper

Professors, Physicians, Healthcare Professionals and the General Public are welcome to use the online interactive whitepaper without charge.

www.Glycosciencewhitepaper.com

The whitepaper in magazine is available in
100 lb high quality glossy stock for training purposes.

Stem Cell Survey

A CD Technical Syllabus

by H. Reg McDaniel, M.D., provided for use by Health care Professionals. There is evidence that Glycomics can increase stem cell proliferation and stem cell function in humans. *Learning and Behavior Problems in Children Responsive to Micro-nutrients Led to Benefits Reported in Infants and Youth and Maternal Alcohol Damage* (FAS). Your contribution of $50 serves as a fund raiser and is shared between The Endowment for Medical Research and the Fisher Institute for Medical Research.

Additional reading and training materials, FREE online support and continuing Glycomics education and research are available.

Readers have access to hundreds of hours of FREE online materials in the form of articles, reports, and video clips. This is a part of the educational effort of The Endowment for Medical Research, Inc.

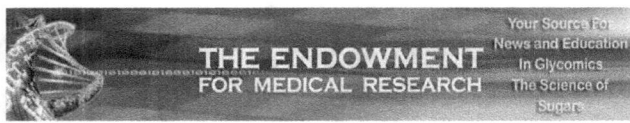

www.endowmentmed.org

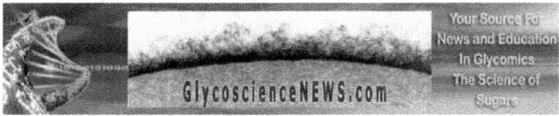

www.GlycoscienceNEWS.com

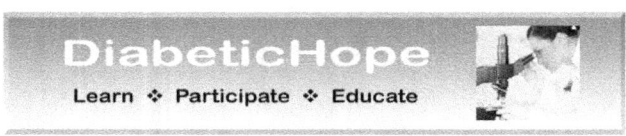

www.DiabeticHope.com

Sources and References:

[1] What You Don't Know About Your Immune System Can Be Deadly Understand your TWO immune systems!
http://www.glycoscienceNEWS.com/pdf/Lesson20.pdf

[2] Improve Your Brain - Expand Your Mind
http://www.endowmentmed.org/pdf/ExpandYourMindImproveYourBrainTableOfContentsCompressed.pdf

[3] http://www.NewsmaxHealth.com/Health-News/ebola-symptoms-spread-early/2014/10/09/id/599812/#ixzz3 Fy3kS0rE

[4] http://fusion.net/video/20107/dr-aileen-marty-tells-fusion-what-she-saw-fighting-ebola-in-nigeria/

[5] http://www.who.int/mediacentre/news/statements/2014/nigeria-ends-ebola/en/

[6] Missing in Action - Why the WHO Failed to Stop Ebola
Time magazine Nov. 10, 2014

[7] http://www.wnd.com/2014/10/if-you-want-to-live-ignore-the-cdc/

[8] http://www.cbn.com/cbnnews/healthscience/2014/October/Doctor-Warns-Test-for-Ebola-Has-One-Fatal-Flaw-/

[9] http://www.wnd.com/2014/10/nyc-has-its-1st-ebola-case/

[10] http://www.dailymail.co.uk/news/article-2806532/So-s-point-NYC-Ebola-patient-PASSED-new-enhanced-screening-JFK-Airport-fall-victim-days-later.html

[11] http://www.wnd.com/2014/10/ebola-victims-without-symptoms-could-still-be-contagious/

[12] http://www.wnd.com/2014/10/who-urges-sneeze-protection-while-cdc-retreats/#U7MEfYlvMK3tBlwS.99

[13] http://www.scientificamerican.com/article/let-s-talk-about-ebola-survivors-and-sex/?WT.mc_id=SA_HLTH_20141104

[14] http://www.afro.who.int/en/clusters-a-programmes/dpc/epidemic-a-pandemic-alert-and-response/outbreak-news/3694-ebola-outbreak-in-democratic-republic-of-congo--update-27-september-2012.html

[15] http://en.mercopress.com/2014/09/12/congo-reports-31-new-ebola-cases-in-the-week-to-9-september

[16] http://radioopensource.org/bausch/

[17] The Hot Zone by Richard Preston - The Most Dangerous Strain page 256

[18] Ibid

[19] http://www.wnd.com/2014/10/move-over-ebola-real-killer-is-coming/?cat_orig=health

[20] http://www.washingtonpost.com/national/health-science/the-ominous-math-of-the-ebola-epidemic/2014/10/09/3cad9e76-4fb2-11e4-8c24-487e92bc997b_story.html

[21] http://www.sfgate.com/news/medical/article/WHO-10-000-new- Ebola -cases-per-week-could-be-seen-5821246.php

[22] Canadian researchers discovered monkeys can catch Ebola from infected pigs without direct contact: http://www.dailymail.co.uk/sciencetech/article-2233956/Could-Ebola-airborne-New-research-shows-lethal-virus-spread-pigs-monkeys-contact.html

[23] http://www.wnd.com/2014/10/is-protective-gear-inadequate-to-stop-ebola/

[24] http://www.scientificamerican.com/article/ebola-spread-shows-flaws-in-protective-gear-and-procedures/?WT.mc_id=SA_TECH_20141014

[25] Ebola contagion in Spain and Germany raises fears for Europe http://news.yahoo.com/eu-demands-explanation-spain-ebola-case-084859314.html

[26] http://hosted.ap.org/dynamic/stories/E/EU_SPAIN_EBOLA?SITE=AP&SECTION=HOME&TEMPLATE=DEFAULT&CTIME=2014-10-06-14-41-22

[27] http://www.wnd.com/2014/10/obama-brings-in-1900-people-from-another-ebola-nation/

[28] http://www.wnd.com/2014/10/panic-hits-home-of-dallas-ebola-victim/

[29] http://latino.foxnews.com/latino/health/2014/10/03/border-patrol-on-alert-after-71-people-from-hard-hit-ebola-countries-illegally/

[30] http://www.Newsmax.com/Newsfront/illegals-immigration-amnesty-executive-order/2014/11/04/id/604991/#ixzz3l6ml0Htd

[31] http://www.americanthinker.com/blog/2014/10/ebola_czar_a_population_control_zealot.html

[32] http://www.dailycollapsereport.com/health/ebola-jihad-terrorists-sicken-thousands/

[33] http://personalliberty.com/ebola-outbreak-advantageous-globalists/

[34] http://fathersforlife.org/health/population_control.htm

[35] http://www.washingtonpost.com/blogs/worldviews/wp/2014/10/24/how-ebola-is-fueling-prejudice-against-gays/

[36] http://www.huffingtonpost.com/g-roger-denson/is-homosexuality-populati_b_784449.html

[37] http://coffee2bsmelt.tumblr.com/post/18016171026/kissinger-eugenics-and-depopulation

[38] http://www.wnd.com/2014/10/is-something-besides-ebola-driving-ebola-epidemic/#DWPSQgDFRvJd3qS4.99

[39] http://www.firstpost.com/world/returning-ebola-medical-workers-should-not-be-quarantined-says-us-cdc-1775539.html

[40] http://www.wnd.com/2014/10/cdc-insists-we-know-how-to-stop-ebola-spread/?cat_orig=health

[41] Non-structural glycoprotein (sGP) papers:
http://www.sciencedirect.com/science/article/pii/S0006291X04018959

[42] http://www.ncbi.nlm.nih.gov/pmc/articles/PMC3094950/

[43] http://jvi.asm.org/content/72/8/6442.full

[44] http://jvi.asm.org/content/79/4/2413.full

[45] http://article.wn.com/view/2014/11/16/Beating_Ebola_Hinged_on_Sipping_a_Gallon_of_Liquid_a_Day/

[46] http://www.bloomberg.com/news/2014-11-16/beating-ebola-hinged-on-sipping-a-gallon-of-liquid-a-day.html

[47] http://freedomoutpost.com/2014/10/us-funds-child-beheading-freedom-fighters-billions-tax-dollars/#4wzVF0ISikPiEw8c.99

[48] http://www.bestofbeck.com/wp/activism/saul-alinskys-12-rules-for-radicals

[49] http://www.wnd.com/2014/10/decorated-combat-troops-sent-to-fight-ebola/

[50] http://yournewswire.com/johns-hopkins-scientist-reveals-shocking-report-on-flu-vaccines/

[51] http://www.wnd.com/2014/10/cdc-lying-to-public-about-ebola-doctor-says/

[52] http://www.wnd.com/2014/10/cnn-savage-has-wild-conspiracy-theories-on-ebola/

[53] http://www.ncbi.nlm.nih.gov/pubmed/7580307

[54] http://www.foxnews.com/us/2012/10/05/rising-career-us-army-officer-matthew-dooley-halted-for-teaching-soldiers-on/

[55] http://www.americanthinker.com/blog/2013/04/pentagon_deep-sixes_lt_col_dooley_for_violating_muslim_pc.html

[56] http://conservatives4palin.com/2014/05/obama-administration-frees-36000-convicted-criminal-aliens-awaiting-deportation.html

[57] http://www.wnd.com/2014/10/obama-plan-to-expose-u-s-to-more-disease/#1tyM3WF12V20djeL.99

[58] http://www.newsmax.com/Finance/Stockman-Fed-central-banks-market/2014/10/22/id/602402/?ns_mail_uid=827494&ns_mail_job=1591896_10232014&s=al&dkt_nbr=ogfd7ijl

[59] http://www.newsmax.com/Finance/Stockman-central-banks-bubble/2014/11/13/id/607258/?ns_mail_uid=827494&ns_mail_job=1595354_11142014&s=al&dkt_nbr=u2dtjyn5

[60] http://snovalleystar.com/2014/05/07/hospital-enlists-robot-for-high-tech-cleaning-chores

[61] http://www.NewsmaxHealth.com/Health-News/Ebola-virus-Xenex-robot/2014/10/13/id/600298/#ixzz3HBwRjRXs

[62] Change Your Sugar - Change Your Life - www.DiabeticHope.com

[63] Ibid

[64] Trehalose reduces cell stress and is an antidepressant http://www.ncbi.nlm.nih.gov/pubmed/23644913

[65] http://www.responsibletechnology.org/gmo-dangers/65-health-risks

Additional supportive educational materials are available:

www.GlycoscienceNEWS.com **SMART SUGARS**

www.OneSmartSugar.com/video.html

Expand Your Mind - Improve Your Brain
http://www.endowmentmed.org/ExpandYourMind/MindEbook3.html

Change Your Sugar, Change Your Life
http://DiabeticHope.com
http://EzineArticles.com/?expert=JC_Spencer

© The Endowment for Medical Research
www.endowmentmed.org.

Free download of the Glycoscience whitepaper
www.Glycosciencewhitepaper.com

Ebola is designed to kill millions!

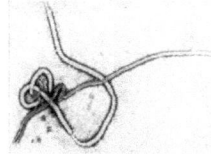

Ebola can cross the oceans in a single bound, just a plane flight away. The bubonic plaque bacteria killed millions in years gone by. Ebola is a serial killer.

Ebola caught humans ill prepared. Politicians disconnected from medical reality may do more harm than good as the embers of the most infectious epidemic smolder under cover of deception.

In a frontal attack on the immune system, Ebola gains a beachhead for victory over humans. With amazing military skill Ebola sets aside the generals of the white blood cell army. It goes straight for the kill by transmitting a message for the cells to surrender their glycoprotein defense system. Within a few days, the human is conquered as structured glycoproteins are fractured into non-structured glycoproteins. These non-structured glycoprotein snippets become the decoys that further confuse the remaining defenders of the immune system.

Billions of dollars are flung at developing new drugs. But, the real answer lies in equipping the existing army of the immune system. Only about 10% of us have an immune system that can kill Ebola. Learn life saving instructions in Ebola Lies.

Some enemies are subtle and some are not so subtle. The purpose we all have is to protect our families from all enemies foreign and domestic. The purpose of **Ebola Lies** is to enable the reader to help save lives and improve individual health. Anything that endangers your life must be exposed and correction.

What you don't know can kill you!

Ebola Lies answers questions the media are not asking and supports the answers with documented evidence.

<u>Ebola Lies</u> separates FACTS from MYTHS.

An educational project of
The Endowment for Medical Research
P. O. Box 73089
Houston, Texas 77273